The Picture World of

Ambulances

Norman Barrett

CONTENTS

Franklin Watts

London • New York • Sydney • Toronto

Introduction

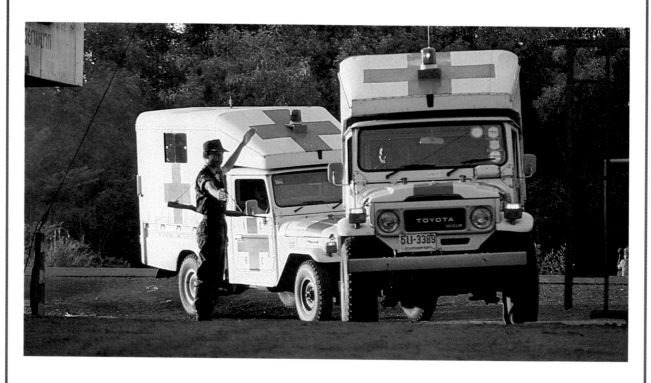

Ambulances are vehicles used mainly for taking sick or injured people to hospital. Modern ambulances carry emergency medical equipment for treating patients on the spot and on the way to hospital. Highly trained ambulance crews, called paramedics, give emergency treatment.

Specially equipped helicopters and planes also serve as ambulances.

△ Red Cross ambulances arrive at a checkpoint in northern Thailand. The Red Cross, an international organization, provides medical help around the world, wherever it is needed.

▷ Inside a typical emergency ambulance. There are two stretchers that serve as temporary beds while the patients are being taken to hospital. First aid equipment includes life-saving apparatus, dressings, splints and medicines.

▽ A helicopter on the scene of a farming accident. Helicopters can fly to and from remote places at great speed.

Emergency ambulances

Emergency ambulances go quickly to where they are needed. They respond to private calls when someone is taken ill in a public place or is injured. Or they may be required to speed to the scene of a major accident or other disaster.

Ambulances have their own central control, which handles emergency calls over a wide area. Control staff are also in contact with the police and fire services.

▽ Police and ambulance crews work together at the scene of a mock-up accident. The two services and the fire brigade co-operate closely during real incidents.

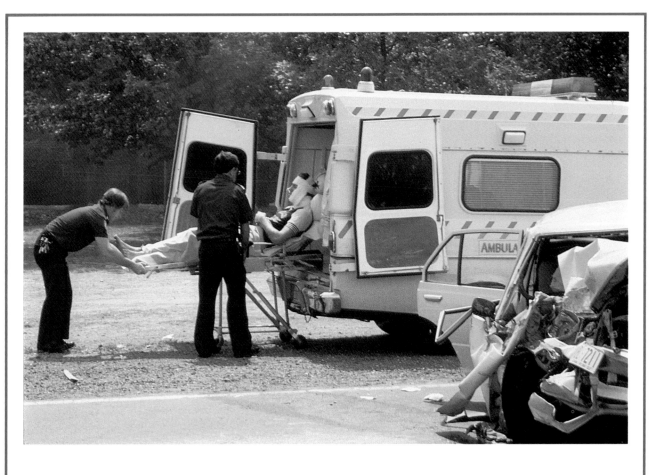

Paramedics give medical treatment to prepare a patient for moving. The equipment they use includes a resuscitator (breathing apparatus), defibrillator (heart machine) and aspirator (suction unit for clearing out the throat). They treat the patient on the way to hospital.

Paramedics may also contact hospital staff, preparing them for the case and perhaps taking advice from hospital doctors.

△ A victim of a road accident is carefully wheeled into an ambulance after being made as comfortable as possible.

9

Most ambulances are purpose-built vans or trucks. They are painted with signs and equipped with flashing lights and sirens, horns or "wailers" to warn other road users to let them pass.

Modern ambulances have two-way radios so that they are in contact with their controls.

Special helicopters are being used more and more for emergency ambulance work.

△ An ambulance based on a Ford Transit chassis, with special bodywork built by another company, Wadham Stringer. The yellow strips are made of material that glows in the dark.

△ Helicopter ambulances operate over areas impossible to reach by road.

▷ A helicopter ambulance with its rear clamshell doors open, showing the amount of medical equipment that can be carried.

◁ Inside the cab of an emergency ambulance, the driver is in touch with the communications center.

▷ Inside, the ambulance is equipped with everything that might be needed in an emergency, including lifesaving drugs and machines to keep patients breathing or regulate their heartbeats.

◁ In some areas, both the driver and the attendant are fully trained paramedics.

Cabinets on the outside of the ambulance store equipment, such as an oxygen cylinder (above) and a stretcher (right).

▷ The modern emergency ambulance is like an operating room on wheels. Instead of side windows, there is storage space both inside and out.

Special ambulances

Some ambulances are built for special purposes, such as for use over rough country or in mountain rescue. Some are converted station wagons or vans, used for taking a single patient on a long journey or quickly between hospitals.

Special ambulances are used by some police departments. Organizations such as the Red Cross also have their own ambulances.

△ An ambulance of the New York City Police Department. Some police forces have their own medical service to treat injured police personnel.

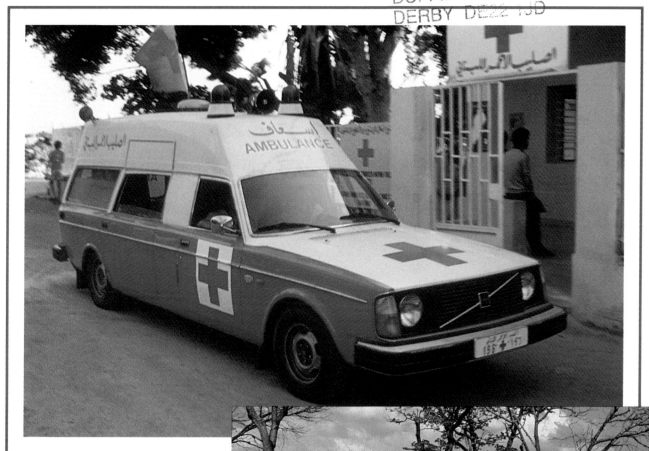

△ An ambulance of the Red Cross, a converted version of a Volvo station wagon.

▷ A van used by the Red Cross as a baby care clinic in Botswana, in southern Africa.

Major incidents

At a major accident with many casualties, a mobile control unit may be set up. This co-ordinates all the ambulance activity and keeps in contact with the other emergency services – police and fire. It also serves as a base for medical teams.

All non-urgent ambulance work in the area is stopped, and extra emergency equipment is brought to the scene.

△ A mobile ambulance control unit (right) at the scene of a major rail crash. This serves as the medical headquarters. It uses radio or direct telephone lines to control all the ambulances and link up with the fire and police services.

16

All areas have special plans for major emergencies, such as rail or plane crashes or natural disasters such as floods or earthquakes.

Extra emergency equipment is brought to the scene in special vehicles. Emergency packs containing everything from hacksaws to hot-water bottles are taken. The usual medical equipment is carried, but with extra blood, oxygen, pain-relieving gas and splints and dressings of all kinds.

▽ Nurses and paramedics attend to survivors of a major train accident as the victims arrive at a hospital. Blood and oxygen continue to be given to a patient.

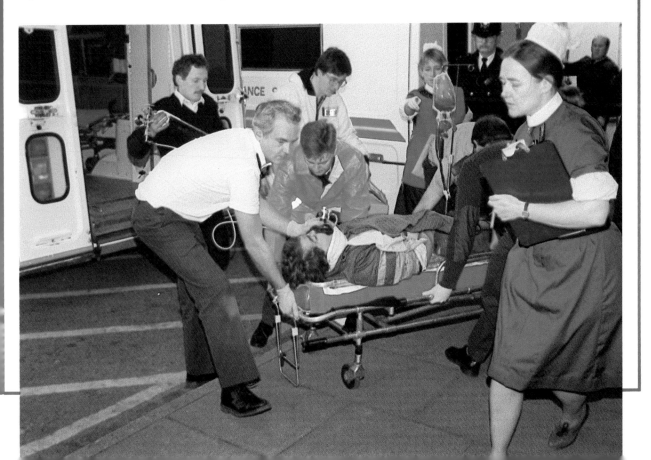

Air ambulances

Aeroplane ambulances can travel long distances quickly and are used for reaching cases in remote areas. Helicopter ambulances are used for carrying patients across the sea or over rough or mountainous country. They can reach difficult places and land almost anywhere.

They are crewed by paramedics and are fully equipped to handle all medical emergencies. Like road ambulances, they keep in contact with medical staff at the hospital.

▷ A patient is wheeled into a helicopter ambulance with paramedics in attendance.

▽ The inside of a flying ambulance has been described as a "mini-emergency room in the sky".

◁ Helicopter ambulances may be used to take crash victims to hospital when roads are blocked with traffic.

Ambulances at war

Wherever fighting takes place, ambulances are needed to move injured troops or civilians away from the battlefield.

Specially equipped ambulances and helicopters are used to take the injured from the "front line" to hospitals and first aid stations away from the fighting.

The Red Cross Society sends its ambulances and medical staff to all parts of the world where they are needed in time of war.

▽ An army ambulance looks out of place on city streets, but they are sometimes used for civilian purposes in emergencies. Military ambulances have to be built like armored cars for battlefield action.

△ Helicopter ambulances are used for evacuating injured soldiers from the battlefield.

◁ A victim of war in Lebanon is treated inside a Red Cross ambulance.

Ambulances on the spot

At big events, where large crowds of people are involved, ambulances wait on standby in case they are needed.

First aid centres at major sporting events, ceremonies or pop concerts deal with minor injuries or illness. But ambulances are always needed in the event of more serious cases to take the patients to hospital.

In some countries, this standby ambulance service is provided by voluntary organizations.

▽ Ambulances on standby at a football match. The St John Ambulance Brigade is a voluntary service providing first aid and emergency ambulances at public events. A British organization, it has spread to other parts of the world.

Transport ambulances

Ambulances are not used just for emergencies. An important part of the work done by ambulance services is the transport of patients.

Patients who find it difficult or impossible to get around by themselves are taken to hospital appointments or day centres for the elderly or handicapped. Many transport ambulances are equipped to carry passengers in wheelchairs.

△ A small ambulance – converted from an estate vehicle – is used for transporting people in wheelchairs. The ramp at the back is raised electrically. Ambulances used for transport work are called "sitting-case" vehicles. Their drivers are not as highly trained as emergency crews.

Facts

The Flying Doctor

Ambulance aircraft are operated by Australia's Royal Flying Doctor Service. They provide an emergency medical service for people living in remote areas – about two-thirds of the continent.

The service has 14 bases across Australia, and is a vital lifeline to more than 100,000 people each year. Without it, many Australians would be faced with a round trip of up to 1,000 km (600 miles) to their nearest doctor.

△ A Flying Doctor aircraft at the Central Australian Aviation Museum. The service has been in operation since 1928.

Fever ambulances

In the last century, people seriously ill in Europe with infectious diseases were taken to the hospital in regular horsedrawn cabs. This put other people using the cabs at great risk of infection. It was not until the 1860s that special carriages were designed for the purpose. These "fever ambulances" were painted inside and had rubber pillows and mattresses so that the whole vehicle could be thoroughly scrubbed and disinfected after each patient.

△ A carriage designed in 1867 for taking fever patients to hospital.

The first ambulances

The first special carriages for the sick were horsedrawn wagons used for transporting injured soldiers in Spain about 500 years ago.

Steam ambulances were first built in 1902, but motorized ambulances began replacing the horsedrawn carriages in 1904.

△ A motorized police ambulance in London in the early 1900s.

The Red Cross
In 1859, a Swiss traveler, Jean Henri Dunant, was horrified to see the suffering of the wounded after a battle in Italy. He formed a group of volunteers to help them, and from this small beginning founded the international Red Cross five years later.

With its headquarters in Geneva, Switzerland, the movement now has societies in more than 130 countries. It provides medical help, equipment, and ambulances in all parts of the world, in both peace and war.

△ A fleet of ambulances of the Cuban Red Cross stand in front of a specially equipped Red Cross plane.

Ambulance in space
A special "ambulance spaceship" may soon be needed. When several astronauts begin to stay in space stations for months at a time, the chances of becoming ill are much greater than with short space flights. The idea of a space ambulance, capable of bringing back astronauts in a matter of hours, is being discussed by scientists planning the new international *Freedom* space station for the late 1990s.

Glossary

Air ambulance
A special helicopter or plane fitted out with the emergency equipment, drugs and dressings necessary to treat patients and keep them alive on the way to hospital. Air ambulances are crewed by paramedics.

Aspirator
A suction pump used for cleaning a patient's throat to restore breathing.

Defibrillator
A machine that applies an electric shock to the chest or heart to restore a patient's regular heart pattern.

Mobile control unit
A vehicle used at major incidents to co-ordinate all ambulance work and medical services and link up with other emergency services.

Oxygen cylinder
Oxygen cylinders provide a supply of oxygen for patients who are having trouble with their breathing. They are used with a resuscitator, which regulates the supply.

Paramedics
Trained ambulance crew qualified to give more than just basic first aid. Paramedics can administer drugs, give injections, and use specialist equipment to keep patients breathing or to regulate their heartbeats.

Resuscitator
Apparatus used to restore and regulate a patient's breathing.

Sitting-case vehicle
Ambulance used for transport work.

Standby
Ambulances wait on standby at big public events, ready to take ill or injured people to hospital.

Stretcher
Equipment used to move a patient who must stay in a lying position to and from an ambulance.

Index

PRINTED IN BELGIUM BY
proost
INTERNATIONAL BOOK PRODUCTION